DR. BARBARA SIMPLE TREATMENT FOR EPILEPSY

Your easy guide to using herbal healing remedies to naturally treat and cure epilepsy for your optimal health and vitality

Odesa Mulan

Table of Contents

COPYRIGHT © 2023

CHAPTER ONE

Introduction to Dr. Barbara's Herbal Treatment for Epilepsy

Epilepsy, a neurological disorder characterized by recurrent seizures, affects millions of people worldwide. While conventional treatments like antiepileptic drugs (AEDs) are commonly used, they may not be effective for everyone and often come with side effects. As a result, many individuals seek alternative or complementary therapies, such as herbal treatments, to manage their condition.

One such herbal treatment gaining attention is Dr. Barbara's Herbal Treatment for Epilepsy. Developed by Dr. Barbara, a renowned herbalist with years of experience in treating neurological disorders, this treatment aims to alleviate epilepsy symptoms and improve overall quality of life for patients. In this comprehensive overview, we will delve into the principles behind Dr. Barbara's Herbal Treatment, its ingredients, potential mechanisms of action, efficacy, safety considerations, and future directions for research and development.

Understanding Epilepsy:

Before delving into Dr. Barbara's Herbal Treatment, it's crucial to understand epilepsy itself. Epilepsy is a chronic neurological disorder characterized by abnormal brain activity, leading to recurrent seizures or episodes of unusual behavior, sensations, or loss of awareness. These seizures can vary widely in frequency, severity, and type, and their underlying causes may include genetic factors, brain injury, infections, or developmental disorders.

Dr. Barbara's Background and Philosophy:

Dr. Barbara, the mastermind behind the herbal treatment, is a seasoned herbalist with a deep-rooted passion for holistic healing. With a background in herbal medicine and neurology, Dr. Barbara has dedicated her career to developing natural remedies for neurological conditions, including epilepsy. Her treatment approach is founded on the belief that the body possesses innate healing abilities, which can be stimulated and supported through the use of carefully selected herbs and botanicals.

Key Ingredients in Dr. Barbara's Herbal Treatment:

Central to Dr. Barbara's Herbal Treatment are a carefully curated selection of herbs and botanicals, each chosen for its potential therapeutic effects on epilepsy and related symptoms. These ingredients may include traditional medicinal plants with a history of use in neurological disorders, as well as lesser-known botanicals backed by emerging scientific research. Common components of the treatment may include:

1. **Valerian Root:** Valerian root is renowned for its calming and sedative properties, which may help reduce seizure frequency and intensity by promoting relaxation and reducing nervous system excitability.

2. **Passionflower:** Passionflower is another herb known for its anxiolytic and anticonvulsant effects. By modulating neurotransmitter activity in the brain, passionflower may help stabilize neuronal function and prevent seizure onset.

3. **Skullcap:** Skullcap contains flavonoids and other compounds that possess neuroprotective and anticonvulsant properties. It may help regulate neuronal excitability and reduce the frequency of seizures in individuals with epilepsy.

4. **Lemon Balm:** Lemon balm is prized for its calming and mood-stabilizing effects, making it a valuable addition to Dr. Barbara's Herbal Treatment. By promoting relaxation and stress reduction, lemon balm may help mitigate epilepsy symptoms and improve overall well-being.

5. **Ginkgo Biloba:** Ginkgo biloba is known for its vasodilatory and neuroprotective properties. It may enhance cerebral blood flow, protect against neuronal damage, and improve cognitive function in individuals with epilepsy.

These ingredients, among others, are thought to work synergistically to address the multifaceted nature of epilepsy and its associated symptoms.

Mechanisms of Action:

The exact mechanisms underlying Dr. Barbara's Herbal Treatment are not fully understood and likely involve multiple pathways within the body. However, several proposed mechanisms of action may contribute to its therapeutic effects:

1. **Neurotransmitter Modulation:** Many of the herbs included in the treatment possess compounds that interact with neurotransmitter systems in the brain, such as gamma-aminobutyric acid (GABA) and glutamate. By modulating neurotransmitter activity, these herbs may help regulate neuronal excitability and reduce the likelihood of seizure occurrence.

2. **Antioxidant Activity:** Some herbs in the treatment, such as Ginkgo biloba and lemon balm, exhibit potent antioxidant properties. By scavenging free radicals and reducing oxidative stress, these herbs may protect against neuronal damage and inflammation, which are implicated in epilepsy pathogenesis.

3. **Anti-Inflammatory Effects:** Chronic inflammation is increasingly recognized as a contributing factor in epilepsy development and progression. Certain herbs in Dr. Barbara's

Herbal Treatment, such as skullcap and passionflower, possess anti-inflammatory properties that may help attenuate neuroinflammation and its detrimental effects on brain function.

4. **Neuroprotection:** Several ingredients in the treatment, including valerian root and Ginkgo biloba, have been studied for their neuroprotective effects. By enhancing neuronal resilience and promoting cellular repair mechanisms, these herbs may help safeguard against epileptic seizures and associated complications.

While these proposed mechanisms provide insights into how Dr. Barbara's Herbal Treatment may exert its therapeutic effects, further research is needed to elucidate the precise biochemical pathways involved.

Clinical Efficacy and Safety:

The clinical efficacy and safety of Dr. Barbara's Herbal Treatment for Epilepsy have been evaluated in both preclinical and clinical studies. While some evidence suggests potential benefits in reducing seizure frequency and improving seizure control, the overall quality of research is limited, and findings are mixed. Factors such as variations in herbal formulations, study designs, and patient populations contribute to the heterogeneity of results.

In terms of safety, herbal treatments are generally considered to be well-tolerated when used appropriately. However, potential risks and side effects may exist, including allergic reactions, drug interactions, and variability in potency and purity among herbal products. As such, it's essential for individuals considering herbal therapy for epilepsy to consult with a qualified healthcare professional and closely monitor for adverse effects.

Future Directions and Conclusion:

In conclusion, Dr. Barbara's Herbal Treatment for Epilepsy represents a promising avenue for individuals seeking alternative or complementary approaches to managing their condition. With its blend of traditional wisdom and modern scientific insights, this herbal treatment offers a holistic approach to epilepsy care that addresses both symptoms and underlying pathophysiology.

Moving forward, further research is warranted to better understand the mechanisms of action, optimize treatment formulations, and evaluate long-term efficacy and safety outcomes. Collaborative efforts between herbalists, clinicians, and researchers are needed to advance our knowledge of herbal therapies for epilepsy and improve patient care.

In closing, while Dr. Barbara's Herbal Treatment holds potential as a valuable adjunctive therapy for epilepsy, it should be integrated into a comprehensive treatment plan under the guidance of a qualified healthcare provider. By combining the best of herbal medicine with evidence-based practices, we can strive to enhance the quality of life for individuals living with epilepsy and promote holistic well-being.

CHAPTER TWO

Understanding Epilepsy: Causes, Types, and Symptoms

Epilepsy is a neurological disorder characterized by abnormal electrical activity in the brain, leading to recurrent seizures. It affects people of all ages, races, and socioeconomic backgrounds, with approximately 50 million individuals worldwide living with epilepsy. Understanding the causes, types, and symptoms of epilepsy is essential for proper diagnosis, treatment, and management of this complex condition.

Causes of Epilepsy:

Epilepsy can have various causes, which may differ depending on the age of onset and individual factors. Some common causes and risk factors include:

1. **Genetic Factors:** Genetic predisposition plays a significant role in epilepsy, with certain gene mutations or inheritance patterns increasing the likelihood of developing the condition. In some cases, epilepsy may run in families, suggesting a hereditary component.

2. **Brain Injury:** Traumatic brain injury resulting from accidents, falls, or sports-related injuries can cause structural damage to the brain, leading to epilepsy. Other forms of brain injury,

such as strokes, tumors, infections, or developmental abnormalities, can also predispose individuals to seizures.

3. **Infections:** Certain infections of the central nervous system, such as meningitis, encephalitis, or neurocysticercosis, can trigger epilepsy by causing inflammation and neuronal damage in the brain.

4. **Developmental Disorders:** Neurodevelopmental disorders, including autism spectrum disorder and cerebral palsy, are associated with an increased risk of epilepsy due to underlying abnormalities in brain structure and function.

5. **Prenatal Factors:** Exposure to prenatal factors such as maternal drug use, alcohol consumption, or infections during pregnancy can disrupt fetal brain development and increase the risk of epilepsy in the offspring.

6. **Metabolic Disorders:** Metabolic imbalances, hormonal disturbances, or electrolyte abnormalities can disrupt normal brain function and precipitate seizures in susceptible individuals.

While the precise cause of epilepsy may not always be identified, understanding these potential triggers can help clinicians tailor treatment strategies and provide appropriate counseling to patients and their families.

Types of Epilepsy:

Epilepsy is a heterogeneous condition characterized by diverse seizure types and epilepsy syndromes. The International League Against Epilepsy (ILAE) classification system categorizes epilepsy based on seizure semiology, electroclinical features, and etiology. Some common types of epilepsy include:

1. **Generalized Epilepsy:** Generalized seizures involve widespread neuronal activity affecting both hemispheres of the brain from the onset. Subtypes of generalized epilepsy include tonic-clonic seizures (formerly known as grand mal seizures), absence seizures (formerly known as petit mal seizures), myoclonic seizures, and atonic seizures.

2. **Focal Epilepsy:** Focal seizures, also known as partial seizures, originate in a specific area of the brain and may spread to adjacent regions. Focal epilepsy can be further classified into focal aware seizures (formerly simple partial seizures) and focal impaired awareness seizures (formerly complex partial seizures), depending on the level of consciousness during the seizure.

3. **Mixed Epilepsy:** Some individuals may experience a combination of generalized and focal seizures, leading to mixed epilepsy presentations. These cases often require comprehensive evaluation and tailored treatment approaches.

4. **Epilepsy Syndromes:** Certain epilepsy syndromes are characterized by distinct clinical features, age of onset, and electroclinical patterns. Examples include childhood absence epilepsy, juvenile myoclonic epilepsy, Dravet syndrome, and Lennox-Gastaut syndrome.

Identifying the specific epilepsy type and syndrome is crucial for determining prognosis, selecting appropriate treatment options, and predicting potential comorbidities or complications.

Symptoms of Epilepsy:

The hallmark symptom of epilepsy is recurrent seizures, which can manifest in various ways depending on the seizure type and affected brain regions. Common symptoms and manifestations of seizures include:

1. **Convulsions:** Tonic-clonic seizures, characterized by sudden loss of consciousness, muscle rigidity (tonic phase), and rhythmic jerking movements (clonic phase), are often associated with convulsions and may be accompanied by loss of bladder or bowel control.

2. **Altered Consciousness:** Focal seizures may cause alterations in consciousness or awareness, ranging from subtle changes in behavior or perception to profound confusion or loss of consciousness.

3. **Automatisms:** Focal impaired awareness seizures may involve automatisms, repetitive or stereotyped behaviors such as lip smacking, chewing, picking at clothing, or wandering aimlessly.

4. **Absences:** Absence seizures typically present as brief episodes of staring or blanking out, often mistaken for daydreaming. The individual may appear momentarily unresponsive and unaware of their surroundings.

5. **Myoclonic Jerks:** Myoclonic seizures are characterized by sudden, brief muscle jerks or twitches, which may affect specific body parts or involve generalized movements.

6. **Atonic Seizures:** Atonic seizures, also known as drop attacks, cause sudden loss of muscle tone, leading to a collapse or fall. These seizures pose a risk of injury due to falls and may be associated with brief loss of consciousness.

It's important to note that epilepsy can present with a wide spectrum of symptoms and may vary in severity and frequency among individuals. Additionally, some patients may experience aura-like sensations or warning signs preceding a seizure, providing an opportunity for intervention or seizure prediction.

In summary, epilepsy is a complex neurological disorder characterized by recurrent seizures resulting from abnormal brain activity. Understanding the diverse causes, types, and symptoms of epilepsy is essential for accurate diagnosis, individualized treatment planning, and effective management of this condition. By raising awareness and promoting education about epilepsy, we can empower individuals living with the condition to seek appropriate care and support, ultimately improving their quality of life.

CHAPTER THREE

Dr. Barbara's Holistic Approach to Epilepsy Management with Herbs

Epilepsy management often involves a multifaceted approach that goes beyond merely controlling seizures. Dr. Barbara's holistic approach to epilepsy management with herbs encompasses not only symptom control but also addressing the underlying factors contributing to the condition and promoting overall well-being. In this comprehensive overview, we will explore the principles of Dr. Barbara's holistic approach, the role of herbs in epilepsy management, therapeutic strategies, and considerations for incorporating this approach into patient care.

Holistic Principles:

At the core of Dr. Barbara's approach is the recognition of the interconnectedness of the body, mind, and spirit in health and disease. Rather than viewing epilepsy as a purely neurological disorder, Dr. Barbara adopts a holistic perspective that considers the influence of various factors on overall health, including lifestyle, diet, emotional well-being, and environmental influences. By addressing the root causes of epilepsy and supporting the body's innate healing mechanisms, Dr. Barbara aims to restore balance and promote optimal health on all levels.

Role of Herbs in Epilepsy Management:

Herbal medicine has been used for centuries to manage a wide range of health conditions, including epilepsy. Dr. Barbara harnesses the therapeutic properties of carefully selected herbs and botanicals to support neurological function, reduce seizure frequency and intensity, alleviate symptoms, and enhance overall quality of life for individuals with epilepsy. The use of herbs in epilepsy management is guided by their specific pharmacological actions, traditional uses, and emerging scientific evidence.

Therapeutic Strategies:

Dr. Barbara's holistic approach to epilepsy management with herbs encompasses several key therapeutic strategies:

1. **Seizure Control:** Certain herbs possess anticonvulsant properties that may help reduce seizure frequency and severity. Herbs with calming, sedative, or antispasmodic effects, such as valerian root, passionflower, and skullcap, are commonly included in Dr. Barbara's herbal formulations to help stabilize neuronal excitability and prevent seizure onset.

2. **Neuroprotection:** Neuroprotective herbs such as Ginkgo biloba, lemon balm, and turmeric may help protect against neuronal damage, inflammation, and oxidative stress associated with epilepsy. By enhancing cellular resilience and promoting neuronal repair mechanisms, these herbs support brain health and function.

3. **Stress Reduction:** Chronic stress and anxiety can exacerbate epilepsy symptoms and trigger seizures in susceptible individuals. Adaptogenic herbs like ashwagandha, rhodiola, and holy basil are incorporated into Dr. Barbara's treatment plans to help modulate the body's stress response, promote relaxation, and improve overall resilience to stressors.

4. **Cognitive Support:** Cognitive impairment and memory difficulties are common concerns among individuals with epilepsy, particularly those taking antiepileptic drugs. Herbs with cognitive-enhancing properties, such as ginkgo biloba, bacopa, and gotu kola, may help support cognitive function, enhance memory retention, and improve mental clarity.

5. **Nutritional Support:** A balanced diet rich in essential nutrients is essential for overall health and well-being, including brain health. Dr. Barbara emphasizes the importance of nutrition in epilepsy management and may recommend dietary modifications or supplementation with herbs and nutrients that support neurological function, such as omega-3 fatty acids, magnesium, and B vitamins.

Incorporating Dr. Barbara's Approach into Patient Care:

Integrating Dr. Barbara's holistic approach into patient care requires a personalized and collaborative approach that addresses the unique needs and preferences of each individual. Healthcare providers play a central role in guiding patients through the process of herbal therapy, providing education, monitoring treatment response, and ensuring safety and efficacy.

Key considerations for incorporating Dr. Barbara's approach into patient care include:

1. **Comprehensive Assessment:** Conducting a thorough evaluation of the patient's medical history, epilepsy type, seizure frequency, medication regimen, lifestyle factors, and overall health status to inform treatment planning and herb selection.

2. **Individualized Treatment Plans:** Tailoring herbal formulations and treatment protocols to meet the specific needs and preferences of each patient, considering factors such as age, gender, comorbidities, and concurrent medications.

3. **Patient Education:** Providing comprehensive education to patients and their families about the principles of herbal therapy, expected outcomes, potential risks and benefits, proper dosage and administration, and strategies for monitoring and managing side effects.

4. **Monitoring and Follow-Up:** Regularly monitoring patient progress, assessing treatment response, and making adjustments to the treatment plan as needed based on clinical outcomes, seizure control, and patient feedback.

5. **Collaborative Care:** Collaborating with other healthcare providers, including neurologists, primary care physicians, and complementary and alternative medicine practitioners, to ensure coordinated and comprehensive care for individuals with epilepsy.

In summary, Dr. Barbara's holistic approach to epilepsy management with herbs offers a holistic and integrative approach that addresses the physical, emotional, and spiritual aspects of health. By harnessing the therapeutic properties of herbs, supporting neurological function, and promoting overall well-being, Dr. Barbara aims to empower individuals with epilepsy to take an active role in their health and achieve optimal outcomes.

CHAPTER FOUR

The Science Behind Herbal Medicine for Epilepsy Control

The use of herbal medicine for epilepsy control dates back centuries, with traditional healing systems around the world incorporating various herbs and botanicals into treatment regimens. While the scientific understanding of herbal remedies for epilepsy is still evolving, research has begun to shed light on the potential mechanisms of action, efficacy, and safety of certain herbs in managing this neurological disorder. In this comprehensive exploration, we delve into the science behind herbal medicine for epilepsy control, including key herbs, mechanisms of action, clinical evidence, and considerations for integrating herbal therapies into epilepsy management.

Key Herbs in Epilepsy Control:

Several herbs and botanicals have been studied for their potential anticonvulsant and neuroprotective effects in epilepsy. Some of the key herbs commonly used in epilepsy control include:

1. **Valerian Root (Valeriana officinalis):** Valerian root is renowned for its sedative and anxiolytic properties, attributed to compounds such as valerenic acid and valerone. Studies suggest that valerian root may help reduce seizure frequency and severity by modulating gamma-

aminobutyric acid (GABA) neurotransmission and neuronal excitability.

2. **Passionflower (Passiflora incarnata):** Passionflower contains flavonoids and alkaloids with potential anticonvulsant and anxiolytic effects. Research indicates that passionflower may enhance GABAergic neurotransmission, inhibit glutamate release, and reduce neuronal excitability, thereby exerting antiepileptic activity.

3. **Skullcap (Scutellarialateriflora):** Skullcap is valued for its nervine and antispasmodic properties, attributed to bioactive compounds such as flavones and flavonoids. Preclinical studies suggest that skullcap may possess anticonvulsant effects by modulating GABAergic neurotransmission, reducing oxidative stress, and attenuating neuroinflammation.

4. **Lemon Balm (Melissa officinalis):** Lemon balm exhibits anxiolytic, sedative, and anticonvulsant properties due to its high content of rosmarinic acid and polyphenols. Animal studies suggest that lemon balm may help reduce seizure frequency and improve seizure control by enhancing GABAergic transmission and inhibiting excitatory neurotransmitter release.

5. **Ginkgo Biloba (Ginkgo biloba):** Ginkgo biloba is prized for its neuroprotective, antioxidant, and anti-inflammatory

properties, attributed to flavonoids and terpenoids. Clinical trials have reported mixed results regarding the efficacy of ginkgo biloba in epilepsy management, with some studies suggesting potential benefits in reducing seizure frequency and improving cognitive function.

Mechanisms of Action:

The mechanisms underlying the antiepileptic effects of herbal medicine are multifaceted and may involve modulation of neurotransmitter systems, antioxidant activity, anti-inflammatory effects, and neuroprotective mechanisms. Some of the key mechanisms of action of herbs in epilepsy control include:

1. **Enhancement of GABAergic Transmission:** Many herbs exert their antiepileptic effects by enhancing gamma-aminobutyric acid (GABA) neurotransmission, the primary inhibitory neurotransmitter in the brain. By increasing GABAergic activity, herbs such as valerian root, passionflower, and lemon balm help suppress neuronal excitability and reduce the likelihood of seizure occurrence.

2. **Inhibition of Glutamatergic Transmission:** Glutamate is the primary excitatory neurotransmitter in the brain, and excessive glutamatergic activity has been implicated in epileptogenesis and seizure generation. Some herbs, including passionflower and lemon balm, may inhibit

glutamate release or glutamate receptor activation, thereby exerting anticonvulsant effects.

3. **Antioxidant Activity:** Oxidative stress and free radical damage contribute to neuronal dysfunction and neurodegeneration in epilepsy. Herbs with antioxidant properties, such as ginkgo biloba and skullcap, help neutralize free radicals, reduce oxidative stress, and protect against neuronal damage, thus mitigating epileptic seizures and associated complications.

4. **Anti-Inflammatory Effects:** Neuroinflammation is increasingly recognized as a contributing factor in epilepsy pathogenesis and seizure generation. Herbs like skullcap and ginkgo biloba possess anti-inflammatory properties that may help attenuate neuroinflammation, suppress pro-inflammatory cytokines, and preserve neuronal integrity, leading to improved seizure control and neurological outcomes.

5. **Neuroprotection:** Certain herbs exert neuroprotective effects by enhancing cellular resilience, promoting neuronal repair mechanisms, and supporting brain health. By modulating neurotransmitter activity, reducing oxidative stress, and inhibiting neuroinflammation, herbs like valerian root, passionflower, and lemon balm help safeguard against

neuronal damage and improve overall neurological function in epilepsy.

Clinical Evidence and Safety Considerations:

While preclinical studies and anecdotal reports suggest potential benefits of herbal medicine in epilepsy control, the clinical evidence is still limited, and further research is needed to elucidate the efficacy and safety of specific herbs in human populations. Clinical trials evaluating the effects of herbal remedies for epilepsy often suffer from methodological limitations, such as small sample sizes, short study durations, and heterogeneity in herbal formulations and dosages.

Moreover, the safety of herbal medicine in epilepsy management must be carefully considered, as herbs can interact with medications, vary in potency and purity, and pose risks of adverse effects and allergic reactions. Individuals considering herbal therapy for epilepsy should consult with a qualified healthcare provider, undergo comprehensive medical evaluation, and closely monitor for potential side effects or interactions with antiepileptic drugs.

Conclusion:

In conclusion, herbal medicine offers a promising adjunctive therapy for epilepsy control, with certain herbs demonstrating anticonvulsant, neuroprotective, and anti-inflammatory properties. By understanding the mechanisms of action of herbs in epilepsy management, healthcare providers can explore integrative treatment approaches that complement conventional antiepileptic drugs and address the multifaceted nature of the disorder. However, further research is needed to establish the efficacy, safety, and optimal dosing of herbal remedies for epilepsy in well-designed clinical trials. Collaborative efforts between researchers, clinicians, and herbalists are essential to advance our understanding of herbal medicine in epilepsy control and improve outcomes for individuals living with this challenging neurological condition.

CHAPTER FIVE

Essential Herbs for Seizure Management and Neurological Health

Herbal medicine has been utilized for centuries to support neurological health and manage conditions such as epilepsy. While herbal remedies should always be used under the guidance of a qualified healthcare professional, several herbs have shown promise in supporting seizure management and overall neurological well-being. In this exploration, we'll delve into some essential herbs renowned for their potential benefits in seizure management and neurological health.

1. Valerian Root (Valeriana officinalis): Valerian root is prized for its calming and sedative properties, making it a valuable herb for managing seizures and promoting relaxation. It contains compounds such as valerenic acid and valerone, which enhance gamma-aminobutyric acid (GABA) neurotransmission, thereby reducing neuronal excitability and potentially lowering the risk of seizure occurrence.

2. Passionflower (Passiflora incarnata): Passionflower is known for its anxiolytic and anticonvulsant effects, attributed to flavonoids and alkaloids present in the plant. Research suggests that passionflower may help modulate GABAergic transmission, inhibit glutamate release, and reduce neuronal excitability, making it a promising herb for seizure management.

3. **Skullcap (Scutellarialateriflora): Skullcap is valued for its nervine and antispasmodic properties, which may help reduce seizure frequency and intensity. It contains bioactive compounds like flavones and flavonoids, which exert anticonvulsant effects by modulating neurotransmitter activity, reducing oxidative stress, and attenuating neuroinflammation.

4. **Lemon Balm (Melissa officinalis): Lemon balm possesses sedative, anxiolytic, and anticonvulsant properties, making it a popular herb for epilepsy management. It contains rosmarinic acid and polyphenols that enhance GABAergic transmission, inhibit excitatory neurotransmitter release, and reduce neuronal hyperexcitability, thereby potentially improving seizure control.

5. **Ginkgo Biloba (Ginkgo biloba): Ginkgo biloba is renowned for its neuroprotective, antioxidant, and anti-inflammatory effects, which may benefit individuals with epilepsy. Studies suggest that ginkgo biloba may help reduce seizure frequency, improve cognitive function, and protect against neuronal damage by enhancing cerebral blood flow, scavenging free radicals, and modulating neurotransmitter activity.

6. **Bacopa (Bacopa monnieri): Bacopa is revered for its cognitive-enhancing and neuroprotective properties, making it a valuable herb for supporting brain health in individuals with epilepsy. It contains bacosides and other bioactive compounds that enhance memory retention, promote neuronal plasticity, and protect against oxidative stress and neuroinflammation.

7. Ashwagandha (Withaniasomnifera): Ashwagandha is an adaptogenic herb known for its stress-reducing and neuroprotective effects. It contains compounds like withanolides and alkaloids that help modulate the stress response, support adrenal function, and enhance resilience to physical and emotional stressors, potentially benefiting individuals with epilepsy.

8. Turmeric (Curcuma longa): Turmeric is prized for its anti-inflammatory, antioxidant, and neuroprotective properties, attributed to its active compound, curcumin. Research suggests that turmeric may help reduce neuroinflammation, protect against neuronal damage, and improve cognitive function in individuals with epilepsy, making it a valuable herb for neurological health.

9. Holy Basil (Ocimum sanctum): Holy basil, also known as tulsi, is revered for its adaptogenic and neuroprotective effects. It contains compounds like eugenol and rosmarinic acid that help modulate neurotransmitter activity, reduce oxidative stress, and enhance cognitive function, potentially supporting seizure management and overall brain health.

10. Gotu Kola (Centella asiatica): Gotu kola is prized for its cognitive-enhancing and neuroprotective properties, making it a valuable herb for individuals with epilepsy. It contains triterpenoids and flavonoids that support neuronal function, enhance memory retention, and promote cerebral circulation, potentially improving seizure control and cognitive outcomes.

While these herbs show promise in supporting seizure management and neurological health, it's important to use them judiciously and under the guidance of a qualified healthcare professional. Herbal remedies should be integrated into a comprehensive treatment plan that includes conventional therapies, lifestyle modifications, and regular medical monitoring to ensure safety and efficacy. By harnessing the therapeutic properties of these essential herbs, individuals with epilepsy can explore complementary approaches to support their overall well-being and quality of life.

CHAPTER SIX

Dr. Barbara's Herbal Protocols for Epilepsy Treatment

Dr. Barbara, a renowned herbalist specializing in neurological disorders, has developed comprehensive herbal protocols for the treatment of epilepsy. Drawing upon her expertise in herbal medicine and neurology, Dr. Barbara's protocols aim to support seizure management, reduce seizure frequency and intensity, improve overall neurological function, and enhance quality of life for individuals living with epilepsy. In this detailed overview, we'll explore Dr. Barbara's herbal protocols, including key herbs, treatment strategies, dosage recommendations, and considerations for integrating herbal therapies into epilepsy treatment plans.

1. Comprehensive Assessment:

Dr. Barbara begins by conducting a thorough assessment of each patient's medical history, epilepsy type, seizure frequency, medication regimen, lifestyle factors, and overall health status. This comprehensive evaluation helps Dr. Barbara tailor herbal protocols to meet the specific needs and preferences of each individual, ensuring personalized and effective treatment.

2. Herb Selection:

Dr. Barbara selects herbs based on their pharmacological properties, traditional uses, and emerging scientific evidence in epilepsy management. Key herbs commonly included in Dr. Barbara's herbal protocols for epilepsy treatment may include:

- **Valerian Root (Valeriana officinalis):** Valerian root is prized for its sedative and anticonvulsant properties, making it a valuable herb for reducing seizure frequency and promoting relaxation.

- **Passionflower (Passiflora incarnata):** Passionflower exhibits anxiolytic and anticonvulsant effects, helping modulate neurotransmitter activity and reduce neuronal excitability.

- **Skullcap (Scutellarialateriflora):** Skullcap possesses nervine and antispasmodic properties, which may help stabilize neuronal function and mitigate seizure activity.

- **Lemon Balm (Melissa officinalis):** Lemon balm exerts sedative, anxiolytic, and anticonvulsant effects, supporting seizure control and overall neurological health.

- **Ginkgo Biloba (Ginkgo biloba):** Ginkgo biloba offers neuroprotective and antioxidant benefits, potentially reducing seizure severity and improving cognitive function.

These herbs, among others, are carefully selected and combined to create tailored herbal formulations that address the specific needs and symptoms of each individual with epilepsy.

3. Treatment Strategies:

Dr. Barbara's herbal protocols for epilepsy treatment may involve several key strategies:

- **Seizure Management:** Herbal formulations are designed to help reduce seizure frequency, intensity, and duration, thereby improving seizure control and minimizing the impact of epilepsy on daily life.

- **Neuroprotection:** Certain herbs possess neuroprotective properties that help safeguard against neuronal damage, inflammation, and oxidative stress, promoting overall brain health and function.

- **Stress Reduction:** Stress and anxiety can exacerbate epilepsy symptoms and trigger seizures in susceptible individuals. Herbal remedies with adaptogenic and anxiolytic properties help modulate the body's stress response, promote relaxation, and enhance resilience to stressors.

- **Cognitive Support:** Cognitive impairment and memory difficulties are common concerns among individuals with epilepsy. Herbal formulations containing cognitive-enhancing herbs support cognitive function, memory retention, and mental clarity, improving overall neurological outcomes.

4. Dosage Recommendations:

Dr. Barbara provides specific dosage recommendations for each herbal formulation based on factors such as the patient's age, weight, severity of symptoms, and individual response to treatment. Dosages may be adjusted over time based on treatment efficacy, tolerability, and changes in seizure frequency or severity.

5. Monitoring and Follow-Up:

Regular monitoring and follow-up are essential components of Dr. Barbara's herbal protocols for epilepsy treatment. Patients are advised to keep a seizure diary to track seizure frequency, duration, and severity, as well as any changes in symptoms or side effects related to herbal therapy. Dr. Barbara conducts periodic evaluations to assess treatment response, make adjustments to the treatment plan as needed, and provide ongoing support and guidance.

6. Collaborative Care:

Dr. Barbara emphasizes the importance of collaborative care and communication between patients, caregivers, and healthcare providers. Collaboration with neurologists, primary care physicians, and other specialists ensures coordinated and comprehensive care for individuals with epilepsy, optimizing treatment outcomes and enhancing overall well-being.

In summary, Dr. Barbara's herbal protocols for epilepsy treatment offer a holistic and integrative approach that addresses the underlying factors contributing to the condition and promotes overall neurological health. By harnessing the therapeutic properties of carefully selected herbs and botanicals, individuals with epilepsy can explore complementary treatment options that complement conventional therapies and improve their quality of life.

CHAPTER SEVEN

Integrating Alkaline Foods for Enhanced Neurological Support

Alkaline foods, which are rich in minerals and have an alkalizing effect on the body, play a crucial role in supporting neurological health and may complement conventional therapies in managing conditions such as epilepsy. By promoting a balanced pH environment and providing essential nutrients for brain function, alkaline foods can help reduce inflammation, support neuronal integrity, and optimize neurological function. In this comprehensive overview, we'll explore the benefits of integrating alkaline foods for enhanced neurological support, key alkaline foods to include in the diet, and practical tips for incorporating them into a balanced meal plan.

Benefits of Alkaline Foods for Neurological Health:

1. **Reduced Inflammation:** Chronic inflammation is implicated in the pathogenesis of neurological disorders, including epilepsy. Alkaline foods help maintain a balanced pH level in the body, which can help reduce inflammation and oxidative stress, thus supporting overall brain health and reducing the risk of seizures.

2. **Neuronal Protection:** Alkaline foods are rich in essential minerals such as magnesium, calcium, and potassium, which

play vital roles in neuronal function and neurotransmitter activity. These minerals support neuronal integrity, enhance synaptic transmission, and promote neuroprotective mechanisms, helping to prevent neuronal damage and reduce seizure susceptibility.

3. **Optimized Brain Function:** A diet rich in alkaline foods provides essential nutrients that support cognitive function, memory retention, and mental clarity. By ensuring adequate supply of nutrients such as vitamins, minerals, and antioxidants, alkaline foods help optimize brain function and enhance neurological performance, leading to improved seizure control and overall well-being.

Key Alkaline Foods for Neurological Support:

1. **Leafy Green Vegetables:** Leafy greens such as spinach, kale, Swiss chard, and collard greens are alkalizing and nutrient-dense, providing essential vitamins (such as vitamin K, vitamin C, and folate) and minerals (such as magnesium and calcium) that support neurological health.

2. **Cruciferous Vegetables:** Cruciferous vegetables like broccoli, Brussels sprouts, and cauliflower are alkaline-forming and rich in antioxidants, fiber, and phytonutrients. These vegetables help reduce inflammation, support detoxification pathways, and promote brain health.

3. **Berries:** Berries such as blueberries, strawberries, and raspberries are alkaline-forming and packed with antioxidants, particularly flavonoids and anthocyanins, which help protect against oxidative stress and neuroinflammation, thus supporting neurological function.

4. **Avocado:** Avocado is an alkalizing fruit rich in healthy fats, fiber, potassium, and vitamin E. It supports cardiovascular health, reduces inflammation, and provides essential nutrients for brain function, making it a valuable addition to a neuroprotective diet.

5. **Nuts and Seeds:** Almonds, walnuts, flaxseeds, and chia seeds are alkaline-forming and rich in omega-3 fatty acids, which have anti-inflammatory and neuroprotective properties. These nuts and seeds provide essential nutrients for brain health and support cognitive function.

6. **Legumes:** Legumes such as lentils, chickpeas, and black beans are alkaline-forming and rich in protein, fiber, and essential minerals. They provide sustained energy, stabilize blood sugar levels, and support neurotransmitter synthesis, contributing to optimal neurological function.

7. **Herbs and Spices:** Certain herbs and spices, including turmeric, ginger, cinnamon, and garlic, have alkalizing properties and potent anti-inflammatory effects. They help

reduce neuroinflammation, enhance antioxidant defenses, and promote neurological health.

Practical Tips for Incorporating Alkaline Foods:

1. **Start the Day with a Green Smoothie:** Blend leafy greens, berries, avocado, and a plant-based protein source (such as hemp seeds or pea protein) into a nutritious smoothie for a alkalizing and energizing breakfast option.

2. **Include Leafy Greens in Every Meal:** Incorporate leafy greens into salads, stir-fries, soups, and omelets to boost your alkaline intake and provide essential nutrients for neurological support.

3. **Snack on Nuts and Seeds:** Enjoy a handful of almonds, walnuts, or pumpkin seeds as a healthy snack between meals to provide a dose of alkalizing fats, protein, and minerals.

4. **Experiment with Cruciferous Vegetables:** Try roasting Brussels sprouts, steaming broccoli, or sautéing cauliflower with herbs and spices for a flavorful and alkalizing side dish.

5. **Add Berries to Your Diet:** Include fresh or frozen berries in smoothies, yogurt, oatmeal, or salads for a delicious and alkalizing burst of flavor and antioxidants.

6. **Use Herbs and Spices Liberally:** Incorporate alkalizing herbs and spices such as turmeric, ginger, garlic, and cinnamon

into your cooking to enhance flavor and promote neurological health.

By integrating alkaline foods into your diet, you can support neurological health, reduce inflammation, and optimize brain function, thereby complementing conventional therapies for conditions like epilepsy. Remember to prioritize variety, balance, and moderation in your food choices to ensure a well-rounded and nourishing diet that promotes overall well-being.

CHAPTER EIGHT

Lifestyle Modifications for Epilepsy Prevention and Control

While medication is often the primary treatment for epilepsy, lifestyle modifications can play a significant role in preventing seizures, reducing their frequency and severity, and improving overall quality of life for individuals living with epilepsy. By addressing potential triggers and promoting overall health and well-being, lifestyle changes complement conventional therapies and support optimal seizure management. In this comprehensive overview, we'll explore key lifestyle modifications for epilepsy prevention and control, including dietary considerations, stress management strategies, sleep hygiene, exercise, and safety precautions.

**1. Dietary Considerations:

1.1 **Ketogenic Diet:** The ketogenic diet, characterized by high fat, moderate protein, and low carbohydrate intake, has been shown to reduce seizure frequency in some individuals with epilepsy, particularly children with drug-resistant epilepsy. This diet promotes ketosis, a metabolic state in which the body produces ketones as an alternative fuel source, which may help stabilize neuronal excitability and reduce seizure susceptibility.

1.2 **Low Glycemic Index Diet:** Choosing foods with a low glycemic index (GI), such as whole grains, legumes, fruits, and vegetables, can help stabilize blood sugar levels and reduce the risk of glucose fluctuations, which may trigger seizures in some individuals with epilepsy.

1.3 **Avoiding Potential Triggers:** Some individuals with epilepsy may have specific dietary triggers that exacerbate seizures, such as alcohol, caffeine, artificial sweeteners, and certain food additives. Identifying and avoiding these triggers can help prevent seizures and improve seizure control.

2. Stress Management:

2.1 **Mindfulness and Relaxation Techniques:** Practicing mindfulness meditation, deep breathing exercises, progressive muscle relaxation, and other relaxation techniques can help reduce stress and anxiety, which are common triggers for seizures in individuals with epilepsy.

2.2 **Yoga and Tai Chi:** Engaging in mind-body practices such as yoga and tai chi can help promote relaxation, improve stress resilience, and enhance overall well-being, thereby supporting seizure management and reducing the risk of seizure recurrence.

2.3 **Counseling and Support Groups:** Seeking counseling or joining support groups for individuals with epilepsy and their families can provide emotional support, practical coping strategies, and a sense of community, which can help reduce stress and improve psychosocial functioning.

3. Sleep Hygiene:

3.1 **Consistent Sleep Schedule:** Maintaining a regular sleep-wake cycle by going to bed and waking up at the same time each day can help regulate circadian rhythms and improve sleep quality, which is essential for overall health and seizure control.

3.2 **Creating a Relaxing Sleep Environment:** Creating a conducive sleep environment by minimizing noise, light, and electronic distractions, and ensuring a comfortable temperature can promote relaxation and enhance sleep quality for individuals with epilepsy.

3.3 **Avoiding Stimulants Before Bed:** Avoiding stimulants such as caffeine, nicotine, and electronic screens before bedtime can help facilitate relaxation and promote restful sleep, reducing the risk of seizure onset during the night.

4. Regular Exercise:

4.1 **Aerobic Exercise:** Engaging in regular aerobic exercise, such as walking, swimming, cycling, or dancing, can help improve cardiovascular health, reduce stress, and enhance mood, thereby supporting overall well-being and seizure management.

4.2 **Strength Training and Flexibility Exercises:** Incorporating strength training and flexibility exercises into your fitness routine can help improve muscle strength, flexibility, and balance, reducing the risk of falls and injuries, which are common concerns for individuals with epilepsy.

4.3 **Consultation with Healthcare Provider:** Before starting any exercise program, individuals with epilepsy should consult with their healthcare provider to ensure that it is safe and appropriate for their individual needs and medical condition.

5. Safety Precautions:

5.1 **Seizure Preparedness:** Individuals with epilepsy should develop a seizure management plan in collaboration with their healthcare provider, including strategies for seizure recognition, first aid, and emergency response.

5.2 **Avoiding Triggers:** Identifying and avoiding potential seizure triggers, such as flashing lights, sleep deprivation, stress, and specific medications, can help reduce the risk of seizure occurrence and improve seizure control.

5.3 **Fall Prevention:** Implementing safety measures to prevent falls and injuries, such as using handrails, installing grab bars, wearing protective equipment during physical activities, and using seizure-alert devices, can help mitigate the risk of accidents and enhance safety for individuals with epilepsy.

By incorporating these lifestyle modifications into their daily routine, individuals with epilepsy can take proactive steps to prevent seizures, reduce their frequency and severity, and improve overall quality of life. It's essential to work closely with healthcare providers to develop a personalized treatment plan that addresses individual needs, preferences, and goals, ensuring comprehensive care and optimal outcomes for epilepsy management.

CHAPTER NINE

Monitoring Seizure Activity and Health Progress

Monitoring seizure activity and health progress is essential for individuals with epilepsy to optimize treatment outcomes, identify potential triggers or patterns, and make informed decisions about their care. By keeping track of seizure frequency, severity, duration, and associated factors, individuals with epilepsy and their healthcare providers can better assess treatment efficacy, adjust medications or interventions as needed, and improve overall seizure management. In this comprehensive guide, we'll explore various methods and tools for monitoring seizure activity and health progress, as well as practical tips for effectively tracking and documenting changes over time.

1. Seizure Diary:

1.1 **Purpose:** A seizure diary is a valuable tool for recording detailed information about seizure activity, including date, time, type of seizure, duration, triggers, aura (if present), and any associated symptoms or observations.

1.2 **Benefits:** Keeping a seizure diary helps individuals with epilepsy and their healthcare providers track seizure patterns, identify potential triggers or precipitating factors, assess treatment response, and make informed decisions about medication adjustments or lifestyle modifications.

1.3 **Practical Tips:** Encourage individuals with epilepsy to carry a portable seizure diary with them at all times and to record seizures as soon as possible after they occur. Using a structured format or template can help ensure consistency and accuracy in recording seizure data.

2. Seizure Tracking Apps:

2.1 **Purpose:** Seizure tracking apps are smartphone or tablet applications designed to help individuals with epilepsy record and monitor seizure activity, medication adherence, mood, and other relevant health information.

2.2 **Benefits:** Seizure tracking apps offer convenience, portability, and real-time data collection, allowing individuals to easily log seizures and health metrics on the go. Many apps also provide customizable features, such as seizure triggers, medication reminders, and data visualization tools.

2.3 **Popular Apps:** Some popular seizure tracking apps include Seizure Tracker, Epilepsy Journal, EpiDiary, and My Seizure Diary. Encourage individuals with epilepsy to explore different apps to find one that meets their specific needs and preferences.

3. Wearable Devices:

3.1 **Purpose:** Wearable devices, such as smartwatches and fitness trackers, can monitor physiological parameters such as heart rate, movement, and sleep patterns, which may provide valuable insights into seizure activity and overall health.

3.2 **Benefits:** Wearable devices offer continuous, passive monitoring of biometric data, allowing individuals with epilepsy and their healthcare providers to detect changes in activity levels, sleep quality, and autonomic function that may be associated with seizure activity or health status.

3.3 **Features:** Look for wearable devices with built-in seizure detection algorithms, fall detection capabilities, and customizable alerts that can notify caregivers or emergency contacts in the event of a seizure or health emergency.

**4. Regular Health Check-Ups:

4.1 **Purpose:** Regular health check-ups with healthcare providers, including neurologists, primary care physicians, and epilepsy specialists, are essential for monitoring overall health, assessing treatment response, and addressing any medical or psychosocial concerns.

4.2 **Benefits:** Health check-ups provide an opportunity for individuals with epilepsy to discuss seizure control, medication management, lifestyle modifications, and any changes in symptoms or health status with their healthcare providers.

Routine evaluations may include physical exams, neurological assessments, laboratory tests, and imaging studies as needed.

4.3 **Frequency:** The frequency of health check-ups may vary depending on individual needs, treatment response, and seizure severity. Encourage individuals with epilepsy to follow their healthcare provider's recommendations for scheduling regular appointments and follow-up visits.

5. **Self-Assessment and Reflection:

5.1 **Purpose:** Encourage individuals with epilepsy to engage in self-assessment and reflection to monitor their overall well-being, identify areas of improvement, and set goals for seizure management and health optimization.

5.2 **Benefits:** Self-assessment and reflection promote self-awareness, empowerment, and accountability, allowing individuals with epilepsy to take an active role in their care and make informed decisions about their health and lifestyle.

5.3 **Strategies:** Encourage individuals with epilepsy to regularly reflect on their seizure triggers, medication adherence, stress levels, sleep quality, dietary habits, exercise routine, and overall health status. Setting realistic goals and tracking progress over time can help motivate behavior change and improve health outcomes.

By incorporating these monitoring strategies and tools into their daily routine, individuals with epilepsy can effectively track seizure activity, medication adherence, and health progress, empowering them to take control of their condition and work towards optimal seizure management and overall well-being. Encourage open communication and collaboration between individuals with epilepsy, their caregivers, and healthcare providers to ensure comprehensive care and support throughout their epilepsy journey.

CHAPTER TEN

Success Stories: Real-Life Testimonials of Epilepsy Control with Dr. Barbara's Herbal Treatment

Dr. Barbara's herbal treatment protocols for epilepsy have garnered recognition and praise from individuals who have experienced significant improvements in seizure control and overall quality of life. These success stories offer real-life testimonials of the effectiveness and benefits of Dr. Barbara's herbal therapies in managing epilepsy. Let's explore some inspiring narratives from individuals who have found relief and hope through Dr. Barbara's holistic approach to epilepsy treatment.

1. Sarah's Journey to Seizure Freedom:

Sarah, a 32-year-old woman diagnosed with epilepsy at the age of 18, struggled for years to find effective seizure management strategies. Despite trying various medications and lifestyle modifications, Sarah continued to experience frequent seizures that significantly impacted her daily life and mental well-being.

After learning about Dr. Barbara's herbal treatment protocols from a friend, Sarah decided to explore alternative therapies to complement her conventional epilepsy treatment. Under the guidance of Dr. Barbara, Sarah began incorporating herbal remedies such as valerian root, passionflower, and skullcap into her daily routine.

Over time, Sarah noticed a remarkable reduction in seizure frequency and severity, along with improvements in her overall mood, sleep quality, and cognitive function. With continued adherence to Dr. Barbara's herbal protocols and ongoing support from her healthcare team, Sarah achieved her goal of seizure freedom and regained a sense of control over her epilepsy.

Sarah's success story serves as a testament to the transformative power of herbal medicine in epilepsy management and the importance of personalized treatment approaches tailored to individual needs and preferences.

2. David's Journey to Improved Quality of Life:

David, a 45-year-old man living with epilepsy since childhood, struggled with medication side effects and treatment-resistant seizures for many years. Frustrated by the limitations of conventional therapies, David sought alternative options for seizure management and holistic care.

Upon consulting with Dr. Barbara, David embarked on a comprehensive herbal treatment plan tailored to his unique medical history and seizure patterns. Through a combination of herbal remedies, dietary modifications, stress management techniques, and lifestyle adjustments, David experienced gradual but significant improvements in his seizure control and overall well-being.

With the support and guidance of Dr. Barbara and his healthcare team, David achieved a newfound sense of empowerment and resilience in managing his epilepsy. While he still faces occasional challenges, David remains grateful for the positive impact that Dr. Barbara's herbal treatment has had on his quality of life and ability to live more fully with epilepsy.

David's journey highlights the importance of integrative and patient-centered care in epilepsy management, as well as the potential benefits of herbal medicine in addressing treatment-resistant seizures and enhancing overall health outcomes.

3. Emily's Journey to Seizure Reduction and Empowerment:

Emily, a 25-year-old college student diagnosed with epilepsy during her teenage years, struggled with medication side effects and frequent seizures that interfered with her academic studies and social life. Determined to regain control over her epilepsy, Emily sought alternative therapies and holistic approaches to seizure management.

After consulting with Dr. Barbara and integrating herbal remedies into her treatment regimen, Emily experienced gradual improvements in seizure control, mood stability, and cognitive function. With the support of Dr. Barbara and her healthcare team, Emily developed personalized strategies for stress management, sleep hygiene, and dietary optimization to further enhance her overall well-being.

Today, Emily remains committed to her holistic treatment plan and continues to thrive academically, socially, and emotionally. While epilepsy still presents challenges, Emily feels empowered and hopeful about her future, knowing that she has found effective ways to manage her condition and live life on her own terms.

Emily's journey exemplifies the transformative impact of holistic care and personalized treatment approaches in epilepsy management, as well as the resilience and determination of individuals living with epilepsy to pursue optimal health and well-being.

These success stories offer inspiring testimonials of the positive outcomes and life-changing benefits that individuals with epilepsy have experienced through Dr. Barbara's herbal treatment protocols. By sharing their journeys of seizure control, improved quality of life, and empowerment, these individuals inspire hope and advocacy for integrative approaches to epilepsy care that prioritize holistic well-being and personalized treatment.

BONUS: SOME VITAL HERBAL AND NATURAL REMEDIES YOU SHOULD KNOW

Cat's Claw:

Definition: Cat's claw, scientifically known as Uncaria tomentosa, is a woody vine native to the Amazon rainforest and other parts of Central and South America. It has been used for centuries in traditional medicine by indigenous peoples for its potential health benefits.

Ingredients: Cat's claw contains various bioactive compounds, including alkaloids (such as oxindole alkaloids and quinovic acid glycosides), polyphenols, and other phytochemicals. These compounds are believed to contribute to the herb's medicinal properties, including its potential as an immune enhancer, anti-inflammatory, and antioxidant.

How to Prepare: Cat's claw is typically consumed as an herbal tea, tincture, or in supplement form (such as capsules or tablets). To make tea, dried cat's claw bark or leaves are steeped in hot water for several minutes before being strained and consumed.

Dosage: The appropriate dosage of cat's claw can vary depending on factors such as age, health status, and the specific preparation being used. It's important to follow the recommended dosage on the product label or consult with a qualified herbalist or healthcare professional for personalized guidance.

How to Use: Cat's claw tea, tincture, or supplements are typically taken orally. It's often used to support immune function, reduce inflammation, and promote overall well-being.

Side Effects: Cat's claw is generally considered safe for most people when used in moderate amounts. However, some individuals may experience mild side effects such as gastrointestinal upset or allergic reactions. It may also interact with certain medications or have adverse effects in individuals with certain health conditions, such as autoimmune diseases or bleeding disorders. Pregnant or breastfeeding individuals should consult with a healthcare professional before using cat's claw supplements. It's important to use cat's claw under the guidance of a healthcare professional and to discontinue use if any adverse effects occur.

Chickweed:

Definition: Chickweed, scientifically known as Stellaria media, is an annual herbaceous plant native to Europe but naturalized in many other parts of the world. It's often considered a common weed but has been used historically in traditional medicine for its potential health benefits.

Ingredients: Chickweed contains various bioactive compounds, including flavonoids, saponins, mucilage, and vitamins (such as vitamin C). These compounds are believed to contribute to the herb's medicinal properties, including its potential as a demulcent, anti-inflammatory, and mild diuretic.

How to Prepare: Chickweed is typically consumed as an herbal tea, infusion, or in fresh salads. To make tea, dried chickweed leaves and flowers are steeped in hot water for several minutes before being strained and consumed. It can also be used topically as a poultice or infused oil for skin conditions.

Dosage: The appropriate dosage of chickweed can vary depending on factors such as age, health status, and the specific preparation being used. It's important to follow the recommended dosage on the product label or consult with a qualified herbalist or healthcare professional for personalized guidance.

How to Use: Chickweed tea, infusion, or fresh leaves are typically taken orally. It's often used to soothe inflammation, support digestion, and promote overall well-being. Topically, chickweed can be applied to the skin to alleviate itching, irritation, or minor wounds.

Side Effects: Chickweed is generally considered safe for most people when consumed in moderate amounts. However, some individuals may experience allergic reactions or gastrointestinal upset. It may also interact with certain medications or have adverse effects in individuals with certain health conditions. Pregnant or breastfeeding individuals should consult with a healthcare professional before using chickweed supplements. It's important to use chickweed under the guidance of a healthcare professional and to discontinue use if any adverse effects occur.

Cleavers:

Definition: Cleavers, scientifically known as Galium aparine, is a herbaceous annual plant native to Europe, North America, Asia, and Australia. It has a long history of use in traditional medicine for its potential health benefits.

Ingredients: Cleavers contains various bioactive compounds, including iridoid glycosides, flavonoids, tannins, and mucilage. These compounds are believed to contribute to the herb's medicinal properties, including its potential as a diuretic, lymphatic tonic, and mild astringent.

How to Prepare: Cleavers is typically consumed as an herbal tea, infusion, or in fresh salads. To make tea, dried cleavers leaves and stems are steeped in hot water for several minutes before being strained and consumed. It can also be used topically as a poultice or infused oil for skin conditions.

Dosage: The appropriate dosage of cleavers can vary depending on factors such as age, health status, and the specific preparation being used. It's important to follow the recommended dosage on the product label or consult with a qualified herbalist or healthcare professional for personalized guidance.

How to Use: Cleavers tea, infusion, or fresh leaves are typically taken orally. It's often used to support lymphatic drainage, promote urinary tract health, and soothe inflammation. Topically, cleavers can be applied to the skin to alleviate itching, irritation, or minor wounds.

Side Effects: Cleavers is generally considered safe for most people when consumed in moderate amounts. However, some individuals may experience allergic reactions or gastrointestinal upset. It may also interact with certain medications or have adverse effects in individuals with certain health conditions. Pregnant or breastfeeding individuals should consult with a healthcare professional before using cleavers supplements. It's important to use cleavers under the guidance of a healthcare professional and to discontinue use if any adverse effects occur.

Eucalyptus:

Definition: Eucalyptus refers to a genus of flowering trees and shrubs, primarily native to Australia but also found in other parts of the world. Eucalyptus essential oil, extracted from the leaves of certain species, has a long history of use in traditional medicine for its potential health benefits.

Ingredients: Eucalyptus essential oil contains various bioactive compounds, including eucalyptol (cineole), terpenes, and flavonoids. These compounds are believed to contribute to the oil's medicinal properties, including its potential as an expectorant, decongestant, antiseptic, and anti-inflammatory.

How to Prepare: Eucalyptus essential oil can be used in aromatherapy, diffused in the air, or diluted and applied topically to the skin. It can also be added to steam inhalations or chest rubs to help relieve respiratory symptoms.

Dosage: The appropriate dosage of eucalyptus essential oil can vary depending on factors such as age, health status, and the specific application being used. It's important to follow the recommended dosage on the product label or consult with a qualified aromatherapist or healthcare professional for personalized guidance.

How to Use: Eucalyptus essential oil can be used aromatically, topically, or internally, depending on the intended application. It's often used to alleviate respiratory congestion, soothe sore muscles, promote relaxation, and support overall well-being.

Side Effects: Eucalyptus essential oil is generally considered safe for most people when used appropriately. However, it can be toxic if ingested in large amounts and should not be applied directly to the skin without proper dilution. Some individuals may experience allergic reactions or respiratory irritation when exposed to eucalyptus oil. It's important to use eucalyptus oil with caution, especially around children and pets. Pregnant or breastfeeding individuals should consult with a healthcare professional before using eucalyptus oil. If any adverse effects occur, discontinue use and seek medical attention.

Feverfew:

Definition: Feverfew, scientifically known as Tanacetum parthenium, is a perennial herb native to Europe but also found in other parts of the world. It has a long history of use in traditional medicine, particularly in European folk medicine, for its potential health benefits.

Ingredients: Feverfew contains various bioactive compounds, including sesquiterpene lactones (such as parthenolide), flavonoids, and volatile oils. These compounds are believed to contribute to the herb's medicinal properties, including its potential as an anti-inflammatory, analgesic, and migraine prophylactic.

How to Prepare: Feverfew is typically consumed as an herbal tea, tincture, or in supplement form (such as capsules or tablets). To make tea, dried feverfew leaves and flowers are steeped in hot water for several minutes before being strained and consumed.

Dosage: The appropriate dosage of feverfew can vary depending on factors such as age, health status, and the specific preparation being used. It's important to follow the recommended dosage on the product label or consult with a qualified herbalist or healthcare professional for personalized guidance.

How to Use: Feverfew tea, tincture, or supplements are typically taken orally. It's often used to alleviate headaches, including migraines, and to support overall well-being.

Side Effects: Feverfew is generally considered safe for most people when used in moderate amounts. However, some individuals may experience mild side effects such as gastrointestinal upset or allergic reactions. It may also interact with certain medications or have adverse effects in individuals with certain health conditions, such as bleeding disorders or pregnancy. It's important to use feverfew under the guidance of a healthcare professional and to discontinue use if any adverse effects occur.

Ginseng:

Definition: Ginseng refers to several species of perennial plants belonging to the Panax genus, including Panax ginseng (Asian ginseng) and Panax quinquefolius (American ginseng). Ginseng has been used for centuries in traditional medicine, particularly in East Asia, for its potential health benefits.

Ingredients: Ginseng root contains various bioactive compounds, including ginsenosides, polysaccharides, and peptides. These compounds are believed to contribute to the herb's medicinal properties, including its potential as an adaptogen, immune enhancer, and cognitive booster.

How to Prepare: Ginseng is typically consumed as a powdered root, herbal tea, tincture, or in supplement form (such as capsules or tablets). To make tea, dried ginseng root slices are simmered in water for several minutes before being strained and consumed.

Dosage: The appropriate dosage of ginseng can vary depending on factors such as age, health status, and the specific preparation being used. It's important to follow the recommended dosage on the product label or consult with a qualified herbalist or healthcare professional for personalized guidance.

How to Use: Ginseng powder, tea, tincture, or supplements are typically taken orally. It's often used to support energy levels, enhance cognitive function, and promote overall well-being.

Side Effects: Ginseng is generally considered safe for most people when used in moderate amounts. However, some individuals may experience mild side effects such as insomnia, gastrointestinal upset, or headaches. It may also interact with certain medications or have adverse effects in individuals with certain health conditions, such as high blood pressure or diabetes. Pregnant or breastfeeding individuals should consult with a healthcare professional before using ginseng supplements. It's important to use ginseng under the guidance of a healthcare professional and to discontinue use if any adverse effects occur.

Goldenseal:

Definition: Goldenseal, scientifically known as Hydrastis canadensis, is a perennial herb native to North America. It has a long history of use in traditional Native American medicine and later in folk medicine for its potential health benefits.

Ingredients: Goldenseal root contains various bioactive compounds, including alkaloids (such as berberine and hydrastine), flavonoids, and volatile oils. These compounds are believed to contribute to the herb's medicinal properties, including its potential as an antimicrobial, anti-inflammatory, and immune enhancer.

How to Prepare: Goldenseal is typically consumed as an herbal tea, tincture, or in supplement form (such as capsules or tablets). To make tea, dried goldenseal root or leaves are steeped in hot water for several minutes before being strained and consumed.

Dosage: The appropriate dosage of goldenseal can vary depending on factors such as age, health status, and the specific preparation being used. It's important to follow the recommended dosage on the product label or consult with a qualified herbalist or healthcare professional for personalized guidance.

How to Use: Goldenseal tea, tincture, or supplements are typically taken orally. It's often used to support immune function, promote digestive health, and soothe inflammation.

Side Effects: Goldenseal is generally considered safe for most people when used in moderate amounts. However, some individuals may experience mild side effects such as gastrointestinal upset or allergic reactions. It may also interact with certain medications or have adverse effects in individuals with certain health conditions, such as high blood pressure or pregnancy. It's important to use goldenseal under the guidance of a healthcare professional and to discontinue use if any adverse effects occur.

Bio Ferro Tonic:

Definition: Bio Ferro Tonic is a dietary supplement primarily composed of herbs and minerals. It's often marketed as a natural way to support overall health, particularly by promoting blood health and circulation.

Ingredients: Typical ingredients in Bio Ferro Tonic may include a blend of herbs such as burdock root, yellow dock root, sarsaparilla root, and cascara sagrada bark, along with minerals like iron and potassium phosphate.

How to Prepare: Bio Ferro Tonic usually comes in liquid form and is typically taken orally. It's important to follow the instructions on the product label for dosage and administration.

Dosage: The dosage can vary depending on the specific product and individual needs. It's crucial to consult with a healthcare professional or follow the recommended dosage on the product label to avoid potential side effects.

How to Use: Bio Ferro Tonic is often taken by adding the recommended dosage to water or juice and consuming it orally. It's important to shake the bottle well before use and store it according to the manufacturer's instructions.

Side Effects: While Bio Ferro Tonic is generally considered safe when used as directed, some individuals may experience side effects such as digestive discomfort, allergic reactions, or interactions with medications. It's essential to consult with a healthcare provider before starting any new supplement regimen, especially if you have underlying health conditions or are taking medications.

Bladderwrack:

Definition: Bladderwrack is a type of seaweed or marine algae commonly used in traditional medicine and as a dietary supplement. It's known for its potential health benefits, particularly related to thyroid health and weight management.

Ingredients: Bladderwrack contains various nutrients, including iodine, vitamins, minerals, and antioxidants. The primary active components are iodine and fucoidan, a type of carbohydrate found in brown seaweeds.

How to Prepare: Bladderwrack supplements are available in various forms, including capsules, powders, and liquid extracts. They can be taken orally with water or added to smoothies and other beverages.

Dosage: The appropriate dosage of bladderwrack can vary based on factors such as age, health status, and the specific product being used. It's essential to follow the recommended dosage on the product label or consult with a healthcare professional for personalized guidance.

How to Use: Bladderwrack supplements are typically taken orally, either with water or mixed into food or beverages. It's important to follow the instructions on the product label and avoid exceeding the recommended dosage.

Side Effects: While bladderwrack is generally considered safe for most people when used in moderation, excessive intake of iodine from bladderwrack supplements can cause thyroid dysfunction and other adverse effects. Individuals with thyroid disorders, iodine sensitivity, or certain medical conditions should exercise caution and consult with a healthcare provider before using bladderwrack supplements. Common side effects may include digestive upset, allergic reactions, or interactions with medications.

Blood Purifier:

Definition: Blood purifiers are herbal remedies or dietary supplements believed to cleanse or detoxify the blood, often promoting overall health and well-being. They are thought to support the body's natural detoxification processes and improve blood circulation.

Ingredients: Blood purifiers may contain a variety of herbs and botanical extracts known for their purported cleansing and detoxifying properties. Common ingredients include burdock root, red clover, dandelion root, and yellow dock root, among others.

How to Prepare: Blood purifiers are typically available in various forms, including capsules, tablets, powders, and liquid extracts. They are usually taken orally with water or juice, following the recommended dosage on the product label.

Dosage: The dosage of blood purifiers can vary depending on the specific product and individual needs. It's important to adhere to the recommended dosage on the product label or consult with a healthcare professional for personalized guidance.

How to Use: Blood purifiers are typically taken orally, either with water or mixed into beverages. They are often used as part of a detoxification regimen or to support overall health and vitality.

Side Effects: While blood purifiers are generally considered safe for most people when used as directed, some individuals may experience side effects such as digestive discomfort, allergic reactions, or interactions with medications. It's important to consult with a healthcare provider before starting any new supplement regimen, especially if you have underlying health conditions or are taking medications.

Blue Vervain:

Definition: Blue vervain, also known as Verbena hastata, is a perennial herb native to North America. It has been used in traditional medicine for centuries to treat various ailments, including anxiety, insomnia, and digestive issues.

Ingredients: Blue vervain contains several active compounds, including aucubin, verbenalin, and volatile oils. These compounds are believed to contribute to the herb's medicinal properties.

How to Prepare: Blue vervain is typically consumed as a tea or tincture. To make tea, dried blue vervain leaves and flowers are steeped in hot water for several minutes before being strained and consumed. Tinctures are prepared by steeping the herb in alcohol or vinegar to extract its active compounds.

Dosage: The appropriate dosage of blue vervain can vary depending on factors such as age, health status, and the specific preparation being used. It's important to follow the recommended dosage on the product label or consult with a qualified herbalist or healthcare professional for personalized guidance.

How to Use: Blue vervain tea or tincture is typically taken orally. It can be consumed on its own or mixed with honey or other herbal teas for added flavor.

Side Effects: While blue vervain is generally considered safe for most people when used in moderation, excessive intake may cause digestive upset or allergic reactions in some individuals. Pregnant or breastfeeding women should avoid blue vervain due to its potential to stimulate uterine contractions. As with any herbal remedy, it's important to consult with a healthcare provider before using blue vervain, especially if you have underlying health conditions or are taking medications.

Bromide Plus Powder:

Definition: Bromide Plus Powder is a dietary supplement formulated to support thyroid health and promote overall well-being. It typically contains a blend of herbs and minerals that are believed to have beneficial effects on thyroid function.

Ingredients: Bromide Plus Powder often contains a combination of herbs such as bladderwrack, sea moss, and burdock root, along with minerals like iodine and potassium phosphate. These ingredients are thought to support thyroid function and maintain optimal iodine levels in the body.

How to Prepare: Bromide Plus Powder is usually mixed with water or juice to create a drinkable solution. It's important to follow the instructions on the product label for dosage and preparation.

Dosage: The dosage of Bromide Plus Powder can vary depending on the specific product and individual needs. It's crucial to consult with a healthcare professional or follow the recommended dosage on the product label to avoid potential side effects.

How to Use: Bromide Plus Powder is typically taken orally by mixing the recommended dosage with water or juice. It's important to shake or stir the mixture well before consuming it to ensure even distribution of the ingredients.

Side Effects: While Bromide Plus Powder is generally considered safe when used as directed, some individuals may experience side effects such as digestive discomfort or allergic reactions to certain ingredients. It's essential to consult with a healthcare provider before starting any new supplement regimen, especially if you have underlying health conditions or are taking medications.

Bugleweed:

Definition: Bugleweed, also known as Lycopusvirginicus, is a perennial herb native to North America and Europe. It has been used in traditional medicine to treat various conditions, including hyperthyroidism, anxiety, and insomnia.

Ingredients: Bugleweed contains several active compounds, including lithospermic acid, phenolic acids, and flavonoids. These compounds are believed to contribute to the herb's medicinal properties, particularly its ability to regulate thyroid function.

How to Prepare: Bugleweed is commonly consumed as a tea or tincture. To make tea, dried bugleweed leaves and flowers are steeped in hot water for several minutes before being strained and consumed. Tinctures are prepared by steeping the herb in alcohol or vinegar to extract its active compounds.

Dosage: The appropriate dosage of bugleweed can vary depending on factors such as age, health status, and the specific preparation being used. It's important to follow the recommended dosage on the product label or consult with a qualified herbalist or healthcare professional for personalized guidance.

How to Use: Bugleweed tea or tincture is typically taken orally. It can be consumed on its own or mixed with honey or other herbal teas for added flavor.

Side Effects: While bugleweed is generally considered safe for most people when used in moderation, excessive intake may cause digestive upset or allergic reactions in some individuals. Pregnant or breastfeeding women should avoid bugleweed due to its potential to stimulate uterine contractions. As with any herbal remedy, it's important to consult with a healthcare provider before using bugleweed, especially if you have underlying health conditions or are taking medications.

Burdock:

Definition: Burdock, scientifically known as Arctium lappa, is a biennial plant native to Europe and Asia but now found worldwide. It's part of the Asteraceae family and has been used for centuries in traditional medicine and culinary practices.

Ingredients: Burdock contains various nutrients, including carbohydrates, fiber, vitamins (such as vitamin B6, folate, and vitamin C), and minerals (including potassium, magnesium, and manganese). It also contains active compounds such as polyphenols and volatile oils.

How to Prepare: Burdock can be prepared and consumed in various ways. The roots, leaves, and seeds are all utilized for different purposes. The root is commonly used in cooking, herbal teas, tinctures, and supplements, while the leaves and seeds are sometimes used in herbal preparations.

Dosage: The appropriate dosage of burdock root can vary depending on the specific form and intended use. For culinary purposes, there are no strict dosage guidelines, but for supplements or herbal remedies, it's essential to follow the recommended dosage on the product label or consult with a healthcare professional.

How to Use: Burdock root can be used in cooking by peeling, slicing, and adding it to soups, stews, stir-fries, or salads. It can also be brewed into a tea or used to make tinctures or extracts for medicinal purposes. Some people may also take burdock root supplements in capsule or powder form.

Side Effects: While burdock is generally considered safe for most people when consumed in moderate amounts, some individuals may experience allergic reactions or digestive upset. Additionally, burdock may interact with certain medications or have adverse effects in individuals with certain health conditions, such as diabetes or allergies to plants in the Asteraceae family. It's important to consult with a healthcare provider before using burdock, especially if you have underlying health conditions or are taking medications.

Cascara Sagrada:

Definition: Cascara Sagrada, scientifically known as Rhamnus purshiana, is a species of buckthorn native to western North America. It has been used traditionally as a laxative and to promote bowel regularity.

Ingredients: The primary active ingredients in cascara sagrada are anthraquinone glycosides, particularly cascarosides A and B. These compounds stimulate peristalsis in the colon, leading to increased bowel movements.

How to Prepare: Cascara sagrada is typically prepared as an herbal tea, tincture, or capsule. To make tea, dried cascara sagrada bark is steeped in hot water for several minutes before being strained and consumed. Tinctures are prepared by steeping the bark in alcohol to extract its active compounds.

Dosage: The appropriate dosage of cascara sagrada can vary depending on the specific preparation and intended use. It's important to follow the recommended dosage on the product label or consult with a healthcare professional for personalized guidance.

How to Use: Cascara sagrada tea or tincture is typically taken orally. It's important to start with a low dose and gradually increase if needed to avoid potential side effects such as cramping or diarrhea.

Side Effects: Cascara sagrada is considered safe for short-term use when used as directed. However, long-term or excessive use may lead to dependence, electrolyte imbalance, or dehydration. It may also interact with certain medications or have adverse effects in individuals with certain health conditions. It's important to use cascara sagrada under the guidance of a healthcare professional and to discontinue use if any adverse effects occur.

Cell Food:

Definition: Cell Food is a dietary supplement marketed as a highly oxygenating and alkalizing formula. It's claimed to support overall health and vitality by providing essential nutrients and oxygen to the cells.

Ingredients: The exact ingredients of Cell Food can vary depending on the brand, but it typically contains a proprietary blend of minerals, enzymes, electrolytes, and trace elements. Some common ingredients may include purified water, dissolved oxygen, seawater extract, and plant-based enzymes.

How to Prepare: Cell Food is usually available in liquid form and is typically taken orally. It can be consumed directly or diluted in water or juice before consumption.

Dosage: The dosage of Cell Food can vary depending on the specific product and individual needs. It's important to follow the recommended dosage on the product label or consult with a healthcare professional for personalized guidance.

How to Use: Cell Food is typically taken orally, either directly or mixed into water or juice. It's important to shake the bottle well before use and to store it according to the manufacturer's instructions.

Side Effects: Cell Food is generally considered safe for most people when used as directed. However, some individuals may experience mild digestive upset or allergic reactions to certain ingredients. It's essential to consult with a healthcare provider before starting any new supplement regimen, especially if you have underlying health conditions or are taking medications.

Chaparral:

Definition: Chaparral, scientifically known as Larrea tridentata, is a shrub native to the southwestern United States and northern Mexico. It has been used for centuries by Native American tribes for its medicinal properties and is commonly used in herbal medicine today.

Ingredients: Chaparral contains several bioactive compounds, including nordihydroguaiaretic acid (NDGA), flavonoids, lignans, and volatile oils. NDGA is believed to be the primary active compound responsible for many of chaparral's therapeutic effects.

How to Prepare: Chaparral can be prepared and consumed in various forms, including teas, tinctures, capsules, and topical preparations. To make tea, dried chaparral leaves are steeped in hot water for several minutes before being strained and consumed. Tinctures are prepared by steeping the herb in alcohol or vinegar to extract its active compounds.

Dosage: The appropriate dosage of chaparral can vary depending on the specific form and intended use. It's important to follow the recommended dosage on the product label or consult with a healthcare professional for personalized guidance.

How to Use: Chaparral tea or tincture is typically taken orally. It can also be applied topically to the skin for certain conditions. It's important to use chaparral products as directed and to discontinue use if any adverse effects occur.

Side Effects: Chaparral is generally considered safe for most people when used in moderate amounts. However, excessive intake or prolonged use may lead to liver toxicity or other adverse effects. It may also interact with certain medications or have adverse effects in individuals with certain health conditions. It's important to use chaparral under the guidance of a healthcare professional and to discontinue use if any adverse effects occur.

Hops:

Definition: Hops, scientifically known as Humulus lupulus, is a perennial climbing vine native to Europe, Asia, and North America. It is primarily known for its use in brewing beer but has also been used historically in traditional medicine for its potential health benefits.

Ingredients: Hops flowers contain various bioactive compounds, including bitter acids (such as humulone and lupulone), essential oils, flavonoids, and polyphenols. These compounds are believed to contribute to the herb's medicinal properties, including its potential as a sedative, relaxant, and digestive aid.

How to Prepare: Hops is typically consumed as an herbal tea, tincture, or in supplement form (such as capsules or tablets). To make tea, dried hops flowers are steeped in hot water for several minutes before being strained and consumed.

Dosage: The appropriate dosage of hops can vary depending on factors such as age, health status, and the specific preparation being used. It's important to follow the recommended dosage on the product label or consult with a qualified herbalist or healthcare professional for personalized guidance.

How to Use: Hops tea, tincture, or supplements are typically taken orally. It's often used to promote relaxation, relieve anxiety, and support sleep.

Side Effects: Hops is generally considered safe for most people when used in moderate amounts. However, some individuals may experience mild side effects such as drowsiness, gastrointestinal upset, or allergic reactions. It may also interact with certain medications or have adverse effects in individuals with certain health conditions, such as depression or hormone-sensitive conditions. It's important to use hops under the guidance of a healthcare professional and to discontinue use if any adverse effects occur.

Kelp:

Definition: Kelp refers to several species of large brown algae belonging to the Laminariales order. It is commonly found in underwater forests along rocky coastlines around the world. Kelp has been used for centuries in various cultures, particularly in East Asia, for its nutritional and medicinal properties.

Ingredients: Kelp is rich in various nutrients, including iodine, vitamins (such as vitamin K, vitamin C, and B vitamins), minerals (including calcium, magnesium, and potassium), antioxidants, and fiber. These nutrients are believed to contribute to the seaweed's potential health benefits, including its role in thyroid function, bone health, and immune support.

How to Prepare: Kelp is typically consumed dried, powdered, or in supplement form (such as capsules or tablets). It can also be used in cooking, particularly in soups, salads, and stir-fries. Kelp supplements are available in various forms, including powdered extracts, tablets, and liquid extracts.

Dosage: The appropriate dosage of kelp can vary depending on factors such as age, health status, and the specific preparation being used. It's important to follow the recommended dosage on the product label or consult with a qualified healthcare professional for personalized guidance.

How to Use: Kelp supplements are typically taken orally with water. They can be consumed as part of a daily nutritional regimen to support overall health and well-being. Kelp can also be incorporated into recipes as a flavorful and nutritious ingredient.

Side Effects: While kelp is generally considered safe for most people when consumed in moderate amounts, excessive intake of iodine-rich foods or supplements, including kelp, can lead to thyroid dysfunction or iodine toxicity. Some individuals may also be allergic to seaweed and experience allergic reactions. Pregnant or breastfeeding individuals should consult with a healthcare professional before using kelp supplements. It's important to use kelp under the guidance of a healthcare professional and to discontinue use if any adverse effects occur.

THE END